MALE & FEMALE SEXUAL/REPRODUCTIVE ORGANS

Descriptions,Stages Of Development, Signs And Functions Of The Reproductive Organs

By

BEATRICE TAYLOR

TABLE OF CONTENT

IV: MALE STAGES OF SEXUAL DEVELOPMENT

V: SIGNS OF SEXUAL DEVELOPMENT IN MALES:

- Body Shape
- Pubic Hair, And Skin Inflammation.
- Penis And Gonad Development
- Wet Dreams And Erections
- Voice Change

VI: THE FEMALE EXTERNAL REPRODUCTIVE ORGANS:

- Labia Majora
- Labia Minora
- Bartholin's Organs
- Clitoris
- Breast

VII: THE FEMALE INTERNAL SEXUAL ORGANS

- Vagina
- Uterus(belly)
- Ovaries
- Fallopian Tubes
- Cervix
- Bartholin's Organs
- Hymen

VII: FEMALE STAGES OF SEXUAL DEVELOPMENT

IX: SIGNS OF SEXUAL DEVELOPMENT IN FEMALE:

- Breast Enlargement
- Pubic Hair
- Vaginal Release
- Periods
- Hips Enlargement
- Ovulation

X: SIMILARITIES AND DIFFERENCES BETWEEN MALE AND FEMALE REPRODUCTIVE ORGANS.

CONCLUSION.

INTRODUCTION

The reproductive system of a living organism, otherwise called the genital framework, is the natural framework comprised of the relative multitude of physical organs associated with sexual proliferation.

The reproductive organ is an assortment of organs and an organization of chemical creation that cooperate to make life.

The male contraceptive framework incorporates the testicles which produce sperm, penis, epididymis, vas deferens, ejaculatory pipes and urethra.

The female contraceptive framework comprises the ovaries which produce eggs or oocytes, fallopian tubes, uterus, cervix, vagina and vulva.

Both the male and female contraceptive frameworks should be working appropriately for a couple to normally imagine. An issue with the construction or capability of either conceptive framework can cause fruitlessness.

THE REPRODUCTIVE/ SEXUAL ORGANS

A reproductive organ (or sex organ) is any essential for a creature or plant that is engaged with sexual multiplication. The regenerative organs together comprise the conceptual framework. In creatures, the **testis** in the male, and the **ovary** in the female, are known as the essential sex organs. All others are called optional sex organs, split between the outer sex organs the privates or outside genitalia, apparent upon entering the world in the two genders and the interior sex organs.

The reproductive organs of a living creature, generally called the genital structure, is the normal system involved the overall huge number of actual organs related with sexual expansion.

The sexual organ is a variety of organs and an association of compound creation that participate to make life.

The male prophylactic system integrates the balls which produce sperm, penis, epididymis, vas deferens, ejaculatory lines and urethra.

MALE REPRODUCTIVE ORGANS

The male reproductive organ is an organization of outer and interior organs that have the capability to create, back, transport, and convey feasible sperm for generation. Prenatally, the male sex organs are shaped affected by testosterone discharged from the fetal testicles; by pubescence, the optional sex organs further create and become practical. Sperm is delivered in the testicles and is moved through the epididymis, ductus deferens, ejaculatory conduit, and urethra. Correspondingly, the fundamental vesicles, prostate organ, and bulbourethral organ produce original liquid that go with and support the sperm as it is discharged from the penis during discharge and all through the treatment interaction.

THE MALE EXTERNAL ORGANS

1: PENIS:

This is the male organ utilized in sex. It has three sections: the root, which appends to the mass of the mid-region; the body, or shaft; and the glans, which is the cone-molded part toward the finish of the penis.

The organ utilized for pee and sex.It has supple tissue which can load up with blood to cause an erection. It contains the urethra, which conveys both pee and semen.

The glans, likewise called the top of the penis, is covered with a free layer of skin called prepuce. This skin is here and there eliminated in a technique called circumcision. The kickoff of the urethra, the cylinder that transports semen and pee, is at the tip of the penis.The glans of the penis likewise contains various delicate sensitive spots.

The body of the penis is round and hollow in shape and comprises three round formed loads. These chambers are made of unique, wipe-like tissue. This tissue contains a huge number of enormous spaces that load up with blood when the man is physically stirred. As the penis loads up with blood, it becomes unbending and erect, which takes into account infiltration during sex. The skin of the penis is free and versatile to oblige changes in penis size during an erection.

2: SEMEN:

which contains sperm (conceptive cells), is removed (discharged) through the finish of the penis when the man arrives at sexual peak (climax). At the point when the penis is erect, the progression of pee is obstructed from the urethra, permitting just semen to be discharged at climax.

Sperm might be minuscule cells, yet they are half answerable for reproduction. Males produce a huge number of these cells every day, yet it takes only one to treat an egg and make a day to day existence.

Sperm is the male regenerative cell or gamete. The expression "gamete" infers that the cell is half of an entirety. At the point when a sperm consolidates with a female gamete, or egg, it brings about a human incipient organism.

3: SCROTUM:

This is the free pocket like sac of skin that hangs behind and beneath the penis it holds the testicles set up. It contains the gonads (likewise called testicles), as well as many nerves and veins.

The scrotum goes about as a "environment control framework" for the testicles. For typical sperm improvement, the testicles should be at a temperature somewhat cooler than internal heat level. Unique muscles in the mass of the scrotum permit it to contract and unwind, drawing the balls nearer to the body for warmth or farther away from the body to cool the temperature.

4: GONADS (TESTICLES):

These are oval organs about the size of huge olives that lie in the scrotum, got at one or the flip side by a design called the spermatic rope. Most men have two testicles. they are a couple of egg-molded organs that protest the scrotum, outwardly of the body. They produce sperm and testosterone, which is the male sex chemical.

The testicles are answerable for making testosterone, the essential male sex chemical, and for creating sperm. Inside the testicles are wound masses of cylinders called seminiferous tubules. These cylinders are liable for creating sperm cells.

THE MALE INTERNAL ORGANS INCLUDES

1: EPIDIDYMIS:

This is a profoundly looped tube that lies at the rear of the testicles. All sperm from the testicles should go through the epididymis, where they mature and begin to 'swim'.

The epididymis is a long, snaked tube that lays on the rear of every gonad. It transports and stores sperm cells that are created in the testicles. It additionally is the occupation of the epididymis to carry the sperm to development, since the sperm that rise out of the testicles are juvenile and unequipped for treatment. During sexual excitement, constrictions force the sperm into the vas deferens.

2: VAS DEFERENS:

This is a thick-walled tube joined to the epididymis. It conveys sperm from the epididymis up to the prostate organ and urethra.

The vas deferens is a long, solid cylinder that moves from the epididymis into the pelvic cavity, to simply behind the bladder. The vas deferens transports mature sperm to the urethra, the cylinder that conveys pee or sperm to beyond the body, in anticipation of discharge.

3: EJACULATORY PIPES:

These are framed by the combination of the vas deferens and the fundamental vesicles. The ejaculatory pipes void into the URETHRA. This is a cylinder that stretches out from the bladder to the outside opening toward the finish of the penis. The urethra conveys both pee and sperm.

The urethra conveys pee from the bladder to beyond the body. In guys, it has the extra capability of discharging semen when the man arrives at climax. At the point when the penis is erect during sex, the progression of pee is hindered from the urethra, permitting just semen to be discharged at climax.

4: FUNDAMENTAL VESICLES:

The original vesicles are sac-like pockets that join to the vas deferens close to the foundation of the bladder. The original vesicles produce a sugar-rich liquid (fructose) that gives sperm a wellspring of energy to assist them with moving. The liquid of the fundamental vesicles makes up a large portion of the volume of a man's ejaculatory liquid, or discharge.

5: PROSTATE ORGAN:

This is a pecan estimated organ that sits in the pelvis. The urethra goes through the center of it. It delivers the liquid emissions that help and sustain the sperm.

The prostate organ is a pecan measured structure that is situated beneath the urinary bladder before the rectum. The prostate organ contributes extra liquid to the discharge. Prostate liquids likewise help to feed the sperm. The urethra, which conveys the discharge to be removed during climax, goes through the focal point of the prostate organ.

6: BULBOURETHRAL ORGANS:

Likewise called Cowper's organs, these are pea-sized structures situated on the sides of the urethra just underneath the prostate organ.These organs produce an unmistakable, tricky liquid that discharges straightforwardly into the urethra.This liquid effectively greases up the urethra and to kill any corrosiveness that might be available because of lingering drops of pee in the urethra.

MALE STAGES OF SEXUAL DEVELOPMENT

Adolescents who were born as male upon entering the world will foster genuinely in specific stages, frequently called Leather expert stages. Your pediatrician or family medical care supplier can figure out what stage your tween or adolescent is at and assume it's normal for their age. The Leather expert stages, alongside rough age ranges, include:

SEXUAL DEVELOPMENT STAGE 1:

The pre puberty stage) The testicles are little and the phallus (penis) is kid-like. There is no pubic hair.

SEXUAL DEVELOPMENT STAGE 2:

- This stage begins From **10 years** of age to **15 years** of age The gonads fill in volume and size.
- The penis has no or slight augmentation.
- The scrotum becomes blushed, more slender, and bigger.

- A couple of pubic hairs become noticeable and they are long, straight, and marginally dim.

SEXUAL DEVELOPMENT STAGE 3:

- Begins From **10 years** of age to **16 years** of age) The testicles keep on filling in volume and size.
- The penis turns out to be longer.
- The scrotum keeps on augmenting.
- Pubic hairs become hazier and curlier and a greater amount of them show up.

SEXUAL DEVELOPMENT STAGE 4:

- From **12 years** of age to **17 years** of age The balls keep on developing.
- The penis keeps on filling long and presently becomes thicker.
- The scrotum becomes bigger and furthermore obscures.
- Pubic hair is coarse, thicker, and wavy like grown-up hair, however there are less hairs than a grown-up has.

SEXUAL DEVELOPMENT STAGE 5:

- The balls are of grown-up size (more noteworthy than 20 ml in volume).
- The scrotum and penis are of grown-up size and structure.
- The pubic hair is of typical grown-up dissemination and volume.

SIGNS OF SEXUAL DEVELOPMENT IN MALES

Males mature somewhat more slowly than females. For individuals allocated male upon entering the world, adolescence starts at **age 11** by and large, albeit beginning as soon as **age 9** or however late as **age 14** seems to be as yet considered normal.

A few guys mature quicker than their companions, and a few actual changes might be more steady than others.

Some of these actual changes are exceptionally private. As a parent, you may not see them, but rather your kid probably will. A portion of these might be humiliating encounters for themselves and they will probably keep a lot of this hidden.

1: BODY SHAPE

Remotely, you might see your kid's body start to develop, yet not long before that occurs, they might put on a little weight and appear as though they're all arms and legs. Next comes a development spray in level, frequently around the period of 13.5

Their shoulders will expand and their muscles will foster more definition, too. They will turn out to be perceptibly more grounded and can exploit that by starting a standard gym routine daily practice whenever wanted.

2: PERSPIRING, HAIR, AND SKIN INFLAMMATION

Individual cleanliness is likely one of the greatest changes for youthful guys. Pre-pubescence, it might have been difficult to inspire them to clean up or scrub down, yet presently they should focus closer on these things as they begin to perspire more and foster stench.

They may before long come to you and get some information about shaving the peach fluff from his face or get some information about antiperspirants. Their chemicals will deliver more oil on their skin and they might be inclined to skin inflammation breakouts.

3: PENIS AND GONAD DEVELOPMENT

The principal indication of pubescence really starts with the development of your child's gonads and scrotum, which will exceed twofold in volume.

Their penis and balls will start to develop as they enter adolescence, as well, as will their pubic hair.

The penis starts by filling long, trailed by width.Around 33% of guys have small magnificent knocks, called papules, on their penises. These knocks seem to be pimples and are ordinary and innocuous, however they are super durable

4: WET DREAM AND ERECTIONS

As your tween or adolescent creates, they might start to have nighttime outflows, or "wet dreams," in which they discharge around evening time while resting. This can happen regardless of a sexual dream and is totally normal.

Conversing with your youngster about nighttime discharges before they happen is useful so they know what's in store and that they didn't coincidentally wet the bed. Tell them that it's simply one more piece of adolescence and that it'll disappear in time.

Compulsory erections are one more huge piece of male adolescence and they can happen whenever, for positively not a great explanation by any means.

5: VOICE CHANGE

Your kid's voice will switch up the time that their development spray has started to dial back a little. This happens in light of the fact that their vocal strings and voice box (larynx) gain mass. as well. Before their voice changes totally, it might break and take off, going from high to low quickly.This can be humiliating for them, so be aware of this.

THE FEMALE REPRODUCTIVE/SEXUAL ORGANS.

The female sexual organ is intended to do a few capabilities.It delivers the female egg cells vital for propagation, called the ova or oocytes. The framework is intended to ship the ova to the site of treatment. Origination, the treatment of an egg by a sperm, typically happens in the tubes.The subsequent stage for the treated egg is to embed into the walls of the uterus, starting the underlying phases of pregnancy. If treatment as well as implantation doesn't occur, the framework is intended to bleed the month to month shedding of the uterine coating. Also, the female regenerative framework produces female sex chemicals that keep up with the conceptive cycle.

THE FEMALE EXTERNAL
REPRODUCTIVE ORGANS

1: LABIA MAJORA:

The labia majora encases and safeguard the other outside contraceptive organs. In a real sense deciphered as "enormous lips," the labia majora are somewhat huge and beefy, and are equivalent to the scrotum in guys. The labia majora contains sweat and oil-emitting organs. After adolescence, the labia majora are covered with hair.

2: LABIA MINORA:

In a real sense deciphered as "little lips," the labia minora can be tiny or up to 2 inches wide. They lie right inside the labia majora, and encompass the openings to the vagina (the channel that joins the lower part of the uterus to the beyond the body) and urethra (the cylinder that conveys pee from the bladder to the beyond the body).

3: BARTHOLIN'S ORGANS:

These organs are situated close to the vaginal opening and produce a liquid (bodily fluid) emission.

4: CLITORIS:

The two labia minora meet at the clitoris, a little, delicate bulge that is practically identical to the penis in guys. The clitoris is covered by an overlay of skin, called the prepuce, which is like the prepuce toward the finish of the penis. Like the penis, the clitoris is exceptionally delicate to excitement and can become erect.

5: BREAST:

The breast are likewise a significant part of the female sexual organ.

At the point when pubescence happens, the female breast creates at a sped up rate because of the impacts of estrogen and other hormones The essential function Trusted Wellspring of the female breast is to deliver milk for breastfeeding. During pregnancy, the chemical prolactin invigorates milk creation, while the chemical oxytocin animates the arrival of milk from the organs. The female breast likewise has a sexual capability, as feeling of the breast or areolas might upgrade delight.

THE FEMALE INTERNAL REPRODUCTIVE ORGANS

1: VAGINA:

The vagina is a waterway that joins the cervix the lower part of the uterus) to the beyond the body. It additionally is known as the birth trench.

2: UTERUS (BELLY):

The uterus is an empty, pear-molded organ that is the home to a creating baby.The uterus is separated into two sections: the **cervix**, which is the lower part that opens into the vagina, and the primary body of the uterus, called the **corpus**. The corpus can undoubtedly grow to hold a creating child. A channel through the cervix permits sperm to enter and feminine blood to exit.

3: OVARIES:

The ovaries are little, oval-formed organs that are situated on one or the other side of the uterus. The ovaries produce eggs and chemicals.

4: FALLOPIAN TUBES:

These are restricted cylinders that are joined to the upper piece of the uterus and act as passages for the ova (egg cells) to make a trip from the ovaries to the uterus. Origination, the preparation of an egg by a sperm, typically happens in the fallopian tubes. The treated egg then, at that point, moves to the uterus, where it inserts into the coating of the uterine wall.

5: CERVIX

The cervix partitions your vagina and uterus, found right between the two. It seems to be a doughnut with a small opening in the center. This opening associates your uterus and your vagina. It lets feminine blood out and sperm in. Your cervix extends open (widens) during labor.

6: BARTHOLIN'S ORGANS

The Bartholin's organs are close to your vaginal opening. They discharge liquid that greases up your vagina (makes it wet) when you're turned on.

7: HYMEN

The hymen is the dainty, plump tissue that stretches across part of the opening to the vagina. Hymens fluctuate a great deal in the amount of your vaginal opening they cover, and they can in some cases (however not generally) tear and cause draining the initial not many times you put something in your vagina.

FEMALE STAGES OF SEXUAL DEVELOPMENT

1: SEXUAL DEVELOPMENT STAGE 1:

Leather expert stage 1 depicts what's befalling your kid before any actual indications of adolescence show up. It regularly begins after a female's eighth birthday celebration and after a male's ninth or tenth birthday celebration. At this stage, these inward changes are no different for guys and females.

The mind starts to convey messages to the body to plan for changes.

The nerve center starts to deliver gonadotropin-delivering chemicals (GnRH) to the pituitary organ, which makes chemicals that control different organs in the body.

Pituitary organ begins to make two different chemicals: luteinizing chemical (LH) and follicle-invigorating chemical (FSH).

Actual changes aren't perceptible for guys or females at this stage.

2: SEXUAL DEVELOPMENT STAGE 2

Stage 2 denotes the start of the actual turn of events. Chemicals start to convey messages all through the body.

Females Adolescence normally begins between ages 9 and 11. Apparent changes include:

- First indications of bosoms, called "buds," begin to frame under the areola. They might be bothersome or delicate or one bud might be bigger than the other, which is typical.
- Hazier regions around the areola (areola) will likewise extend.
- Uterus starts to get bigger, and modest quantities of pubic hair begin developing on the lips of the vulva.

3: SEXUAL DEVELOPMENT STAGE 3

These changes in females start after age 12. These progressions include:

- Bosom "buds" proceed to develop and extend.
- Pubic hair gets thicker and curlier.
- Hair begins shaping under the armpits.

- The main indications of skin break out may show up on the face and back.
- The most noteworthy development rate for level starts (around 3.2 inches each year).
- Hips and thighs begin to develop fat.

4: SEXUAL DEVELOPMENT STAGE 4

In females, stage 4 generally begins around age 13. Changes include:

- Bosoms take on a more full shape, passing the bud stage.
- Numerous females get their most memorable period, commonly between ages of 12 and 14, yet it can happen prior.
- Level development will dial back to around 2 to 3 inches each year.
- Pubic hair gets thicker.

5: SEXUAL DEVELOPMENT STAGE 5

- Bosoms arrive at surmised grown-up size and shape, however bosoms can keep on changing through age 18.

- Periods become ordinary following a half year to 2 years.
- Females arrive at grown-up level 1 to 2 years after their most memorable period.
- Pubic hair finishes up to arrive at the inward thighs.
- Conceptive organs and private parts are completely evolved.
- Hips, thighs, and posterior finish up in shape.

SIGNS OF SEXUAL DEVELOPMENT IN FEMALES

1: BREAST ENLARGEMENT

Young ladies for the most part start pubescence between the ages of 8 and 13 years of age. The earliest indication of adolescence in many young ladies is the improvement of bosom "buds," nickel-sized knocks under the areola. It is entirely normal for bosom development to begin on one side before the other. It's likewise normal for breast buds to be fairly delicate or sore. Lopsided breast development and touchiness are both absolutely typical and ordinarily improve with time.

2: PUBIC HAIR

Coarser hair will start to fill in the genital region, under the arms, and on the legs. In certain young ladies (around 15%), pubic hair might be the primary indication of puberty showing up before bosom sprouting begins.

3: VAGINAL RELEASE

A few young ladies experience a little direct measure of clear or white vaginal release that begins around 6 a year prior to their most memorable period. This is an ordinary reaction to developing measures of the chemical estrogen in the body.

4: PERIODS

Menstruation, or period, is typical vaginal draining that happens as a feature of a lady's month to month cycle. Consistently, your body gets ready for pregnancy. Assuming no pregnancy happens, the uterus, or belly, sheds its covering. The feminine blood is halfway blood and part of the tissue from inside the uterus. It drops off the body through the vagina.

Periods typically start between age 11 and 14 and go on until menopause at about age 51. They generally last from three to five days.

While courses of events can change, most young ladies get their most memorable period inside 2 - 3 years after the improvement of breast buds.

5: HIPS ENLARGEMENT

Frequently, the hips enlarge, the abdomen turn out to be relatively more modest, and additional fat is created around the stomach and rear end. Yet, all bodies grow contrastingly during this time, and there is no "typical." Every individual fosters their exceptional size and shape.

6: OVULATION

Ovulation is a piece of your monthly cycle. It happens when an egg is set free from your ovary.

At the point when the egg is delivered, it could conceivably be fertilized by sperm. Whenever treated, the egg might make a trip to the uterus and embed to form into a pregnancy. On the off chance that is left unfertilized, the egg crumbles and the uterine covering is shed during your period.

Understanding how ovulation occurs and when it happens can help you accomplish or forestall pregnancy.

SIMILARITIES BETWEEN MALE AND FEMALE REPRODUCTIVE ORGANS

- Both Male and female reproductive organs are liable for the creation of gametes, preparation, and the improvement of the incipient organism into another person.
- The two frameworks are situated around the pelvic district.
- They produce gametes.
- Barrenness, contaminations, tumors, immune system issues, and hereditary anomalies are the illnesses related with the two sorts of regenerative frameworks.

DIFFERENCES BETWEEN MALE AND FEMALE REPRODUCTIVE ORGANS.

Male reproductive organs	Female reproductive organs
Intended for the conveyance of sperms into the female reproductive organ.	Intended for supporting a child
Most parts happens outside the body	Each part happens inside the body
Parts: penis, scrotum, original vesicle,vas deferens,Prostate , and Cowper's organ	Parts: vulva, clitoris, vagina, cervix, uterus, fallopian tubes, ovaries,and mammary organs

Testicles are the male gonads	Ovaries are female gonads
Male Urethra conducts both pee and semen	Female Urethra happens independently from the vagina opening.
Produce GnRH,LH,FSH,and testosterone	Produces GnRH,LH,FSH, progesterone and estrogen.
Male have a persistent creation of chemicals	Females have a cycle of creating chemicals which causes periods.
Capabilities: creation and conveyance of sperm into female reproductive organ.	Capabilities: produces ova, gets sperms,facilitating treatment and supporting and sustaining the developing embryo.

Constantly delivers gametes.	Creation of gametes stops at menopause .
Produces one billion sperms each month.	Produces a solitary ovum each month

CONCLUSION

The reproductive organs are one of the most important and delicate parts of the human body,the Male reproductive organs are obviously different from that of the female organs, and the two need each other to reproduce younger ones, the Male organs can't reproduce on their own without the female organs.

Made in the USA
Monee, IL
05 March 2023

29147799R00024